OUR MOTHER NATURE

YOUR NATURAL FOOD SOURCE FOR HEALING

James A. York

ISBN: 9781718071346

First Print Edition: 08 2018

Content

INTRO

BURDOCK

DANDELION

ELDERBERRY

LAMBS QUARTER

MULLEIN

STINGING NETTLE

OREGANO

SPEARMINT

SUMAC (RHUS CORIARIA)

WILD CARROT

WILD LETTUCE

WOOD SORREL

MIXING HERBS

DISCLAIMER

Intro

The information in this book belongs to all of us, forgotten knowledge we all once knew. There was a time man and woman could name every plant on their property, telling you the uses and benefits. To understand our natural food is to understand that we are electrical and the only substance that complements us is electrical, the only electrical substances are a product of creation mother nature herself.

Naturally we are all brothers and sisters from Mother Nature she nutritious all on this planet and she did not turn her back on us we turned are back on her and yet she has never stopped providing.

From the beginning of time man and woman are brought into this world by a woman, their mother.

Just like the birds in the sky, land animals and fish in the water. We all follow our mother for the first bit of our lives we do what she does and eat what she eats, we need to re-enter this cycle.

I believe in that there is only one

disease, Dr. Otto Warburg said "no disease can live in an alkaline environment" now with any disease the mucus membrane has been compromised by an acid substance here are some examples

if it is Pneumonia mucus is covering the cells of the lungs, if it's bronchitis there is mucus obstructing the bronchial tubes, or sinus sidise then the mucus is obstructing the nasal passage, mucus is even the problem with aids it's in the skin, blood and lymphatic system that makes up the immunological system.

Our body is alkaline and our food

should be alkaline.

Let's look at animals in captivity they get disease their diet has changed, they don't get their natural food in their natural surroundings. The same animals in the wild do not get disease however they can fall ill, but they correct this by chewing on certain plants.

Getting into un-natural and natural plants all that is natural is on the alkaline side of the ph. scale the molecular structure is complete. The ph. scale is numbered 1 to 14 with 7 being neutral 6.9 and below is acid no signs of life, the molecular structure is incomplete. 7.1 And higher is alkaline it's electrical, it's alive and the molecular structure is complete complementing the human body. Naming a couple of un-natural plants, aloe Vera, carrots and some natural ones are burdock, wild yams, queen's Ann's lace. An un-natural plant is made by man by cross breeding a combination of natural plants and for good intention, to have a plant yield more produce. The problem that is over looked is the molecular structure is incomplete; the un-natural plant is not electrical. Here is an example of cross breeding; the wild yams were crossed with queen's Ann's lace (wild carrot) to make the orange carrots we are all familiar with. When you look at the roots of these plants you will see the wild yam and wild carrot have a much longer root system and the orange carrots in our gardens don't have a long root system. This is another way of knowing natural and un-natural plants, the root system of the natural plant go deep into the earth reaching the mineral level allowing it to absorb much more nutrients and minerals. None of the plants in our gardens that we are familiar with have a long root system but their natural ancestors in the wild do. Just think pick any plant we are familiar with in our gardens and tell me where in the world would I find that plant in the wild, you just won't. There have been studies to see if man was gone from earth how long it would take wood structures to be gone and how long for the steel ones, well what about our gardens? It would be a year or two and it would be gone, because they are not alive, they are not electrical. Without man to intervene they would just die off but not their natural ancestors they will always be here just like they always have been.

This manipulation goes beyond plants it's the animals to and it's nothing new it has gone on for thousands of years. I don't want to get too much into the animals but I'll point out one and some reasoning. The pig, where in the world would I find the pig we are all familiar with that we get are bacon from? You won't, you will find the ancestor of the modern day pig the wild boar. But what farmer wants to raise a bunch of wild boars it would be much easier if they had no tusks, no hair. And let the cross breeding, gene manipulation begin. Once again if man was gone from the planet in just a few years so would the pig. Not the wild boar he will still be here.

From the beginning of time two things have played a big role in society and dividing man more than any other, God and science. So I wanted to bring them both in on this, God teaches that the herbs are for the healing of a nation. Science shows the human body is carbon base and you have to have a carbon base substance to compliment it.

Chemical infinity is an electrical transfer that proves the human body can only accept what it is made of not something new or alien to it. Also the father of medicine (Hippocrates), now before Hippocrates if one got sick it was blamed on the gods. Hippocrates was the first to observe his patients, diagnose and treat, he established the first medical schools all with herbs no chemicals. Hippocrates was known for curing all sickness with herbs. Some might be familiar with a quote from Jane Goodall "How could we have ever believed that it was a good idea to grow are food with poison", well I can imagen Hippocrates saying How could we have ever believed that it was a good idea to put chemicals in our herbs (Medicine).

Addressing sickness and disease, I start with an intracellular cleansing cleaning the cells of toxin that brought the sickness or disease on in the first place. Removing meat, lactose, carbonic acid and uric acid this prevents mucus buildup and creates an alkaline environment. Then by building the body back up with natural energy by using the natural plants.

Dr. Otto Warburg said "No disease can live in an alkaline environment ". He is the man who discovered the cause of cancer and won the noble prize for it then went on to write a book on how to cure cancer and won a second noble prize.

No disease can live in an alkaline environment, like a fish can't live in an environment without water. Wright now we are on a highly acidic diet and disease can thrive, we need to change our diets. When we come to an understanding that when are creator of all that is natural does things they need to be respected. Here is a small list of natural plants.

Burdock

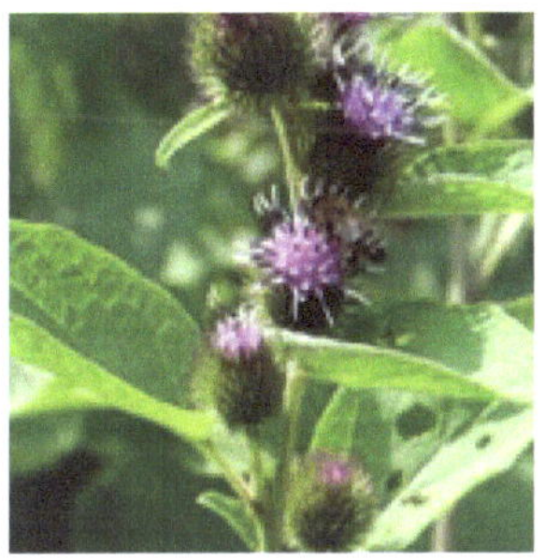

It's full of carbohydrates, fatty oils, plant sterols, tannins, and volatile oils. Studies have shown that burdock contains phenolic acids, quercetin, and lutein, which are all powerful antioxidants. Burdock Root contains vitamins A, E and proper amounts of electrolyte potassium and low in sodium. Potassium is an important component that helps control heart rate and blood pressure. Also it contains some valuable minerals iron, manganese, magnesium; and small amounts of zinc, calcium, selenium, and phosphorus. It is the dried root of burdock that has been mostly used in Tea, soup, salads and capsules for a blood purifier it increases urine flow kills germs and reduces fever. It has also been used to treat cancer, joint pain, bladder infection and acne.

Dandelion

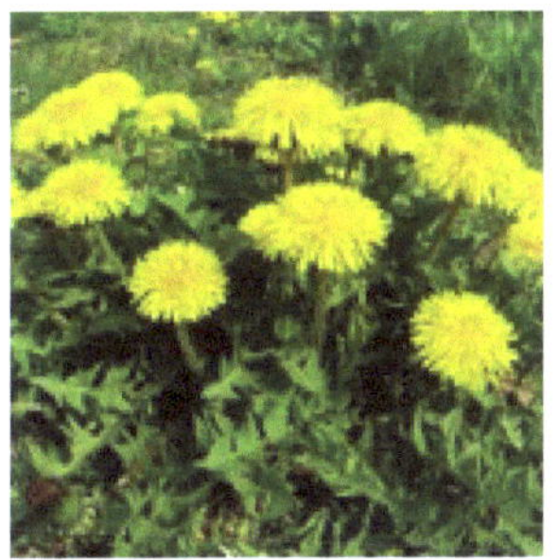

Roasted coffee, okay it's really tea, but because of the dark brew and even the smell some people refer to it as coffee. No caffeine and is super healthy for you and has become one of my favorite drinks hot or cold and could possibly replace coffee for me.

Find some dandelions free of pesticides cut off the roots. Wash the roots real good chop the roots into small pieces and roast. When they finish roasting you can boil in water for 4 or 5 min then strain and enjoy. Health benefits are digestion improves, aids in weight loss will ease congestion of the liver. Helps to purify the bladder and kidneys reduce the risk of urinary tract infection. Helps to ease the bloating, aching joints and can cure skin conditions. Also it helps to purify the blood and regulate blood sugar levels improves overall blood circulation It Contains vitamins B and C, calcium,

magnesium, iron, zinc and potassium.
This is on the alkaline side of the PH
scale.

ELDERBERRY

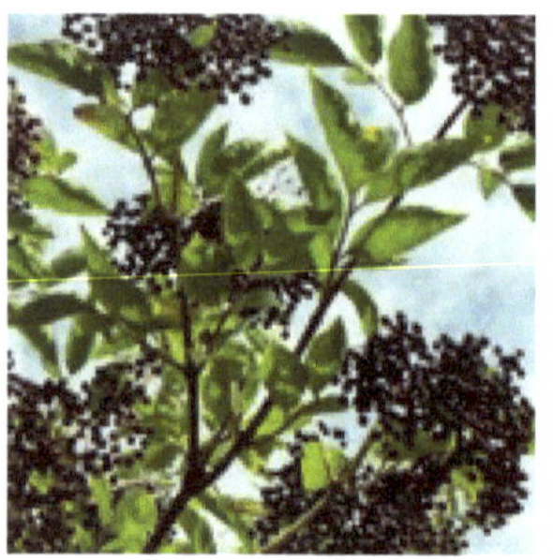

One cup of fresh berries contains approximately 73 calories, 18.4 grams of carbs and less than 1 gram each of fat and protein Vitamin C, dietary fiber and antioxidants in the form phenolic acids, flavonols and anthocyanins. The flowers are rich in flavonols. It's been used for the flu, swine flu, HIV/AIDS, and boosting the immune system. It is also used for back and leg pain, nerve pain, and chronic fatigue syndrome.

Horsetail

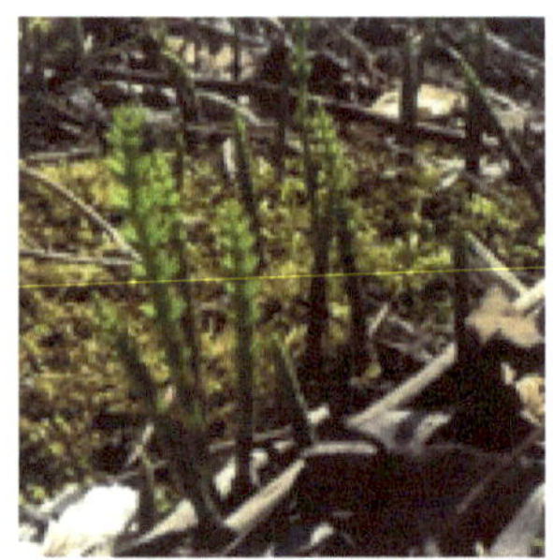

A nutritious herb high in minerals

Removes toxic aluminum from our body with the silica this plant produces. Strengthens bones and fingernails helps hair growth

Horsetail can be crushed into powder for cooking or boiled for tea. When consumed the silica go's through the intestinal wall into your blood stream and binds with aluminum witch is a Nero toxin that actually promotes dementia and Alzheimer. Aluminum enters our body from food we eat, over the counter medication and even vaccines. With the aluminum binding to the silica our kidneys can now flush this toxin from our body.

Lambs Quarter

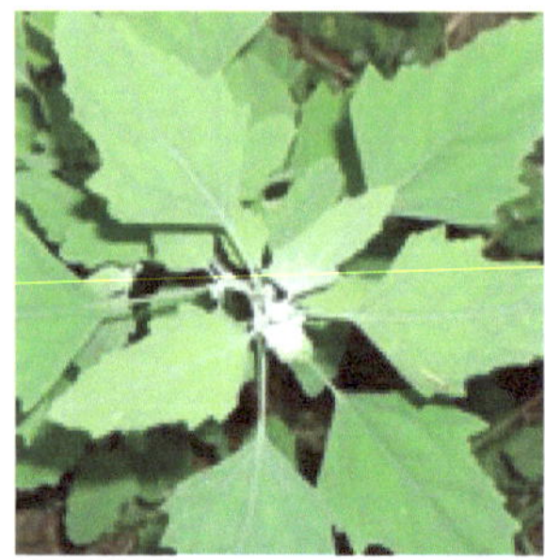

Use as a spinach substitute, salads, stir fry, soups, and you can grind seeds into dark flour to make bread also dried leaves make delicious flour, mix with a bit of water to make tortillas.

Lambs Quarter contains Protein, Carbohydrates, Calcium, Potassium, Beta Carotene, Niacin, and Iron. It is high in vitamin A, and phosphorus it's also a good source of protein, trace minerals, B-complex vitamins, vitamin C, and are extremely essential for normal functioning of the body organs as well as heals long term illness.

All parts of the plant can be used as a poultice arthritis and swelling. For toothaches chewing the lambs' quarter will help. Capsules make a super good vitamin.

Mullein

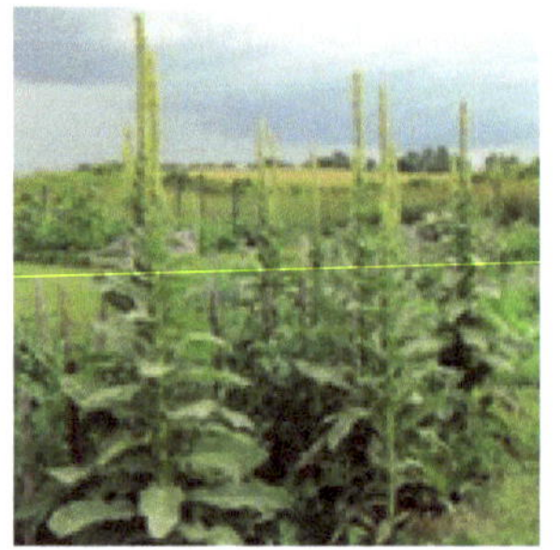

There are over 40 active compounds most notable are Coumarin and glycosides in addition to the minerals, potassium, calcium, iron, magnesium, manganese, phosphorous, and selenium.

Mullein is an expectorant that induces removal of phlegm and mucous from the lungs, it was used to treat respiratory disorders this is just one of its many medicinal uses.

Benefits of mullein include treatment for tuberculosis; it is known that mullein contains expectorant and bacterial properties. Drinking mullein will help with cold or flu with a lot of congestion, allergies, asthma and bronchitis. Mullein is a natural anti-inflammatory, anti-bacterial and anti-spasmodic. Drinking mullein helps with digestive problems like diarrhea, constipation, hemorrhoids, and bladder infections.

Some of the common way to use mullein, you can use the leaf and flowers for tea fresh or dried. The fresh flowers can be used in salad or a smoothie. The leaf can be dried and smoked, even when smoked it soothes inflamed or infected lungs and will prevent coughing. The oils from the flower can be extracted and works against ear infections.

Stinging nettle

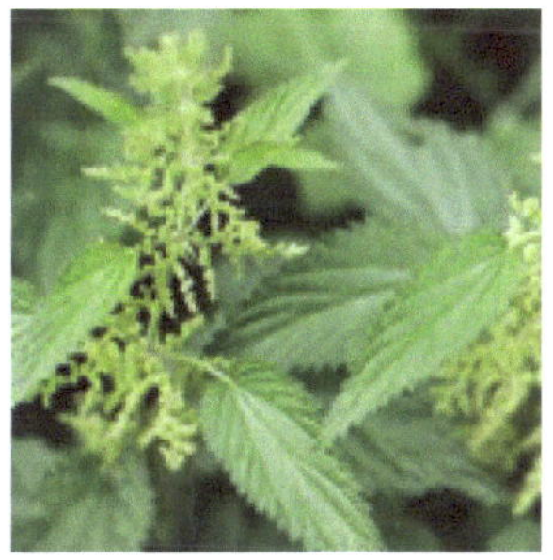

Nettle has a variety of beneficial uses, not just medicinal and a food source but a fertilizer to. Nettle has a high content of vitamins A, B2, C, K, Iron, Potassium, Manganese and even Calcium. It contains up to 25% protein. Nettle is useful in expelling gravel from the bladder and dissolving kidney stones. The herb is a powerful blood purifier that drives out toxins and metabolic wastes by stimulating the kidneys to excrete more water. The tea from Nettle herb will clean out the entire intestinal tract while activating the body's natural defense mechanisms. The tea will also kill and expel intestinal worms. The stinging nettle is proven to relief the symptoms of Rheumatism and Arthritis, some studies point that nettle helps reduce sneezing and itching in Hay Fever sufferers and also helps clean the blood. Because of the vitamins it contains, stinging nettle helps to treat the symptoms of Colds & Flu.

A strong infusion (tea) is helpful in the treatment of dysentery, diarrhea, hemorrhoids and inflammation of the kidneys. It is also useful in the treatment of asthma since it helps expel phlegm from the lungs.

Nettle leaf: when steeped and drunk regularly the tea can help regulate the levels of acetylcholine produced by the adrenal glands. (Acetylcholine is one of the principal neurotransmitters whose levels in the body are affected by nicotine use)

Nettle Fertilizer:

The nutrients in stinging nettle fertilizer are the same nutrients the plant contains like minerals, essential amino acids, proteins and vitamins. A nettle leaf plant food will have: Chlorophyll Nitrogen Iron Potassium Copper Zinc Magnesium Calcium These nutrients, along with Vitamins A, B1, B5, C, D, E, and K, combine together to create a tonic and immune builder for the garden.

How to Make:

Steep 1 ounce of nettles in 1 cup of boiling water for 20 minutes to an hour, then strain the leaves and stems out and toss in the compost bin. Dilute the fertilizer 1:10 and it's ready for use.

Using Nettles as Fertilizer:

One part fertilizer to 10 parts water for watering plants or 1:20 for direct foliar application Undiluted mix makes an excellent organic herbicide

and can be added to the compost bin
to stimulate decomposition.

Note: some plants, like tomatoes and
roses, do not like the high iron levels
in nettle fertilizer.

This fertilizer works best on leafy
plants and heavy feeders. Start with
low concentrations and move on.

I almost forgot, yes you can smoke it
to. It has a reputation for being a
strong and stimulating smoking herb.

OREGANO

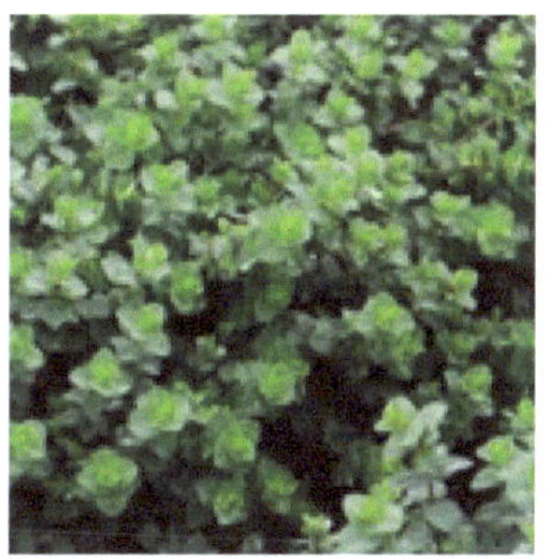

Rich in fibre, iron, copper, magnesium, zinc, potassium, manganese, calcium, and vitamins C, E and K In addition, it contains antioxidants and antibacterial properties. It's been used for treating respiratory tract disorders, gastrointestinal disorders, menstrual cramps, and urinary tract disorders Also rheumatoid arthritis, headaches, heart conditions and fatigue.

Spearmint

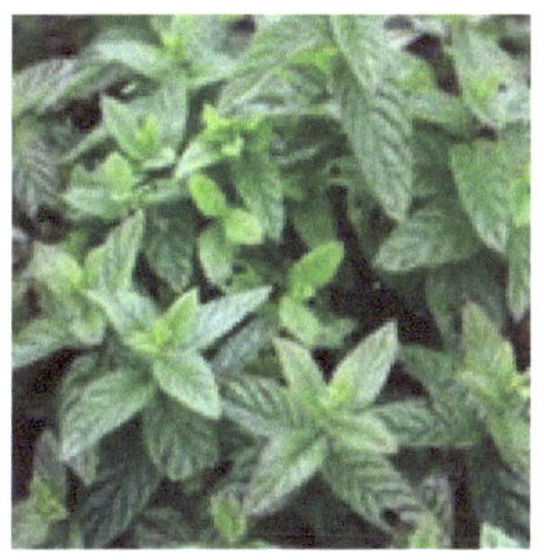

Active ingredients menthol, flavonoids, Mint L-carvone (responsible for odor), potassium, calcium, manganese, iron and magnesium It's been used to alleviate symptoms of nausea, indigestion, gas, headache, toothache, cramps, and sore throat.

Spearmint is refreshing in iced beverages. Spearmint has a wide range of applications, flavor sauces, dips, dishes, or hygienic products, toothpaste, mouthwashes, soaps, and body scrubs. Spearmint tea is perhaps the most direct and beneficial.

The natural antibacterial and antimicrobial nature of menthol and other organic compounds in spearmint help protect your mouth and throat from infections.

Spearmint tea has a significant impact on the health of your respiratory system due to its naturally soothing and anti-inflammatory qualities.

The high iron content can stimulate the production of red blood cells and hemoglobin. Also increases circulation to the body's extremities, boosting energy levels and healing wounds.

The high potassium levels found in spearmint help maintain healthy blood pressure, it relieves the stress on blood vessels and arteries, therefore helps prevent atherosclerosis, strokes, and heart attacks.

Sumac (Rhus coriaria)

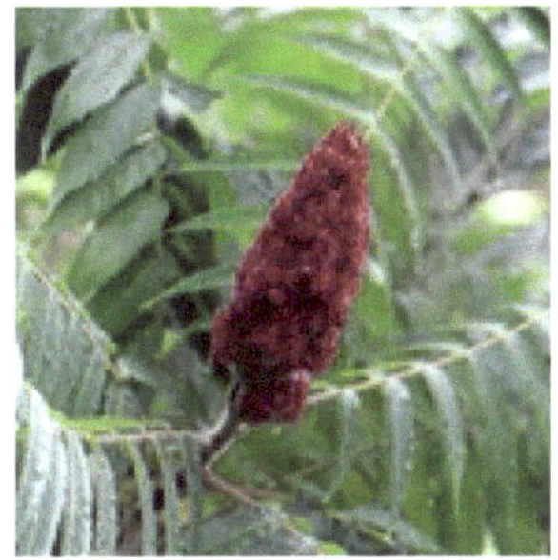

The herb is rich in citric acid, potassium, calcium and magnesium Also malic acid, tannic acid and Gallic acid.

The berries of the Sumac are used to

reduce fever. An infusion mixed with honey makes an herbal cough syrup.

The berries of sumac possess anti-fungal actions against human pathogens.

Sumac berries are considered a powerful anti-inflammatory, applied externally to treat skin inflammatory conditions and arthritis also used to purify blood and to treat sore throat. Lowers bad cholesterol, while boosting good cholesterol

The sumac has become one of my

favorites; I like to use the berries. Fresh or dried they can be made into hot and cold beverages. I like to make a runny jelly so I can pour it on my cereal, ice cream or even a salad and it's easy to add to a smoothie.

WILD CARROT

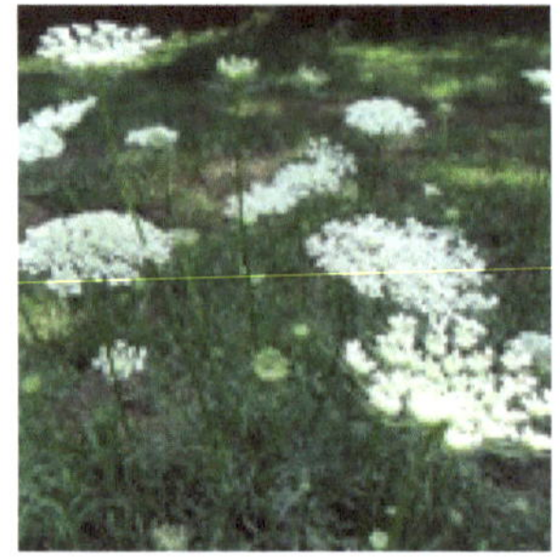

The herb consists of beta-carotene and other properties that are used to treat bladder and kidney conditions. Highly nutritious, Carrots are a particularly good source of beta-carotene, fiber, vitamin K, potassium and antioxidants. They are a weight

loss friendly food and have been
linked to lower cholesterol levels.

Wild Lettuce

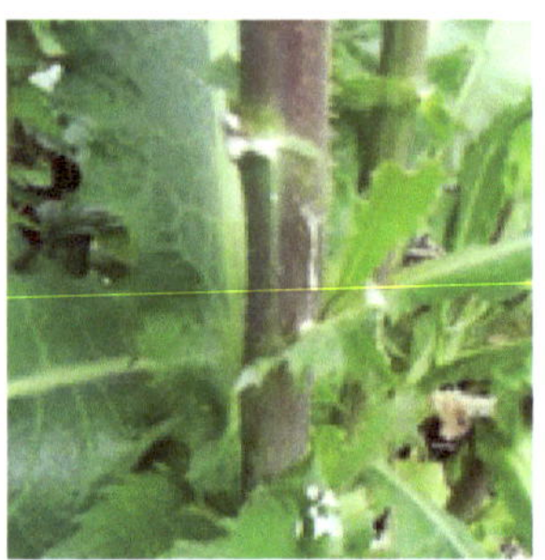

Active compounds in wild lettuce are lactupicrin, lactucin and lactucopicrin.

Nutritional value of wild lettuce
100% Beta Carotene, Calcium,

Magnesium, Sodium, Vitamin A, B, C

The milky fluid from wild lettuce is Lactucarium. Wild lettuce has been called Opium lettuce do to its sedative properties and reports of mild euphoria, similar to morphine. However wild lettuce contains no opiates and has no addictive properties.

The wild lettuce has been used for menstrual pain, increasing the flow of milk in a nursing mother, migraines, urinary tract problems, joint pain, stress, excessive sex drive, asthma, cough, colic, anxiety, restlessness, insomnia.

The common ways of using the wild lettuce, I like them all. If you like leaf lettuce instead of iceberg lettuce then you will love the wild lettuce on your burgers or sandwiches and in a salad, I love adding it to a smoothie. The leaf can be dried for tea or smoked, wild lettuce is a smoke able herb. And by boiling the wild lettuce in water only you can extract the oils for smoking.

Two chemicals responsible for the

properties of wild opium lettuce;

lactucopicrin:

A bitter substance that has a sedative and analgesic effect, acting on the central nervous system

lactucin:

A bitter substance that forms a white crystalline solid It has been shown to have analgesic and sedative properties.

Wild lettuce has opioid-like effects.
Yet, it has none of the addictive
properties of true opioids.

Wood sorrel

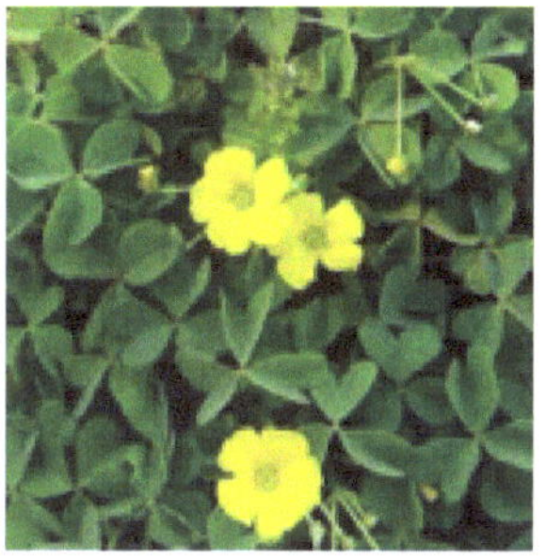

Wood sorrel has a rich, sour, lemony flavor. High in iron, calcium, fiber, magnesium, potassium, vitamin C and A also high in oxalic acid.

Some of its beneficial properties are

diuretic properties, fever reduction, increasing appetite and reducing inflammation when applied.

The iron in sorrel boosts the red blood cell production and prevent anemia (iron deficiency).

Iron is the only mineral that is magnetic it attracts all the other minerals to it so when you ingest iron you are ingesting all minerals. Iron revitalises the cells in the blood and conveys oxygen to the brain and oxygen is what the brain converts and uses for electricity.

Mixing Herbs

Capsule Herbs:

To prepare capsules, simply grind the dried roots, leaves or blooms of the plant and fill capsules with the powder.

Poultices:

Plant material mashed, which is applied externally so that the herb's properties can be absorbed by the skin. Used to reduce inflammation, improve circulation and speed the healing of cuts, scrapes and other sores.

Tinctures:

Soak fresh or dried ground herbs in alcohol to extract and preserve the active compounds of the plant. An advantage of tinctures is that it has a long shelf life.

Making essential oils:

Using olive oil, just fill your jar with the herb pour your oil in seal it tight place in a cool dark location for 4 to 6 weeks

Coconut oil is a very effective way to extract and preserve the active compounds of the plant due to its high saturated fat content. It is capable of absorbing much more than butter or other oils. Coconut oil a saturated fat its chock full of health promoting properties and is in no way responsible for high cholesterol, obesity, heart disease In fact, it's quite the opposite. We're only beginning to uncover the amazing health benefits and you know what else these health benefits are evidence-based. In addition to the three I listed earlier, there is research to support that coconut makes you less hungry, contains ketones that reduce seizures, improves blood cholesterol, burns fat, and boosts brain function in Alzheimer's patients.

Warm your coconut oil in a crockpot with a cup of water never heating more than 110 Celsius put your herb in let simmer 4 to 6 hours strain well pour into a bowl let harden in fridge. The oil will separate from the water hardening at the top. Take the oil off and discard the water and you're done. If you wanted you can use a double boiler to warm and pour into containers of choice.

DISCLAIMER

The following copy provides general information on health topics only for educational and informational purposes as part of a general discussion of public health. It is not medical advice, diagnosis, opinion, treatment or service to you or any other persons and is not a substitute for medical care. Never disregard professional medical advice or delay seeking it because of this copy. Please make sure to ask your physician or other health care provider to assist you in understanding any information you may obtain from this copy or any other sources.

You can cross-reference any information in this copy from witch I sourced.

Massachusetts Institute of technology

(M.I.T),

Yale,

Harvard,

Medical science center

(MSC),

Hippocrates

(Father of Medicine),

Dr. Otto Warburg

(Discovered the cause of cancer and wrote a book on how to cure it winning him two Nobel prizes).

Dr. Sebi

(Claimed to cure cancer aids and more, he was charged with fraud brought before a superior court judge and won his case representing himself).